Cause for Concern

CAUSE *for* CONCERN

POEMS BY
Carrie Shipers

WINNER OF THE 2014 ABLE MUSE BOOK AWARD

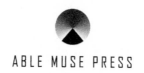

ABLE MUSE PRESS

Able Muse Press

www.ablemusepress.com

Printed in the United States of America

Library of Congress Control Number: 2015940920

ISBN 978-1-927409-59-6 (paperback)
ISBN 978-1-927409-60-2 (digital)

Cover image: "On Visiting" by Alexander Pepple

Cover & book design by Alexander Pepple

Able Muse Press is an imprint of *Able Muse:* A Review of Poetry, Prose & Art—at www.ablemuse.com

Able Muse Press
467 Saratoga Avenue #602
San Jose, CA 95129

For Randal

Acknowledgments

I am grateful to the editors of the following journals where many of these poems originally appeared, sometimes in slightly different forms.

32 Poems: "John Wayne."

Able Muse: "Argos," "In Certain Light," "Aftermath."

Alaska Quarterly Review: "At the Sadness Factory," "He Watches the Weather Channel."

Borderlands: Texas Poetry Review: "The Absence of Trees."

Cimarron Review: "When you embark on a catastrophe."

Conclave: A Journal of Character: "Love Poem to a Murder Ballad," "Wind Rattling the Stalks."

Connecticut Review: "Letter from a Place I've Just Arrived."

Descant: "Without Our Noticing or Being Much to Blame."

The Fiddleback: "The History of Dogs."

Georgetown Review: "The Rapture."

Harpur Palate: "Dear Hospital."

The Hiram Poetry Review: "The Notion of Dog."

The Gettysburg Review: "Self-Portrait as Donald Crowhurst."

Kestrel: "Carry," "Heaven," "Trade Agreement."

Mid-American Review: "How Sandbag Lives Up to His Name."

Midwestern Gothic: "In your next letter," "Instructions for Surviving Slow Apocalypse."

New England Review: "Anti-Anxiety Poem," "Prayer to Our Lady of Waiting Rooms," "Wound Assessment."

New Letters: "Love Poem to Ted Neeley in *Jesus Christ Superstar.*"

Paddlefish: "The Dogs of Malta," "Expedition's End."

Paterson Literary Review: "Home Health."

Permafrost: "Voice of God."

Poet Lore: "Migration," "Self-Portrait as Aerialist. "

The Southern Review: "Confession," "*Fidelis.*"

Tar River Poetry: "Undone."

"Love Poem to Ted Neeley in *Jesus Christ Superstar*" was reprinted in *American Life in Poetry;* "Confession" was reprinted on *Verse Daily.*

Thank you to Alex Pepple and Able Muse Press for making such a beautiful book, and to Molly Peacock for selecting the manuscript. Thank you to Andrea Scarpino, who read every first draft and without whom this book wouldn't exist, and to Hilda Raz, a continual source of wisdom, encouragement, and humor. Thank you to all the friends who sustained me, especially emily m. danforth, Pat Emile, Kelly Grey Carlisle, and Cousin Satchel. As always, thank you to my parents, who knew I'd be a poet before I did. I also wish to thank the University of Nebraska-Lincoln and my brilliant colleagues at the University of Wisconsin Colleges.

Foreword

WHEN WE VISIT THAT FOREIGN COUNTRY known as illness, we are tourists who learn the uncomfortable language of charts and bandages, pills prescribed at certain times of the day. We speak visiting hours and prognosis. We become adept in the customs of this culture, learn to expect casseroles and flowers at first, then later silence from friends and family who wonder how long before they can leave. If illness is a country inhospitable to guests, then Carrie Shipers's second poetry collection, *Cause for Concern,* is our guidebook, preparing us for what we will find in the waiting room, by the bedside, in the bathroom, or on the skin when the gauze is lifted.

In the book's opening poem, "Wound Assessment," a speaker describes binding her husband's wound, a scene dark with the shadows of Caravaggio's paintings. The husband is pierced, almost holy in his pain, and the wife anguished in her knowledge that agonies can't be forgotten. "Even if we fall out of love,/ divorce and never speak again," she explains, "we'll still know/ each other's wounds—his on the left/ like Christ's, mine invisible and aching." And in "Prayer to Our Lady of Waiting Rooms," the hospital becomes a site of pilgrimage and prayer. "Let the news/ be good or benign," pleads the speaker, the country of illness not a land of miracles but of modest hopes. "[L]et us walk outside feeling better,/ or at least no worse, than we did before." There are letters too, as when the poet writes "Dear Hospital," grief transformed into hate mail: "I hate your smell of potatoes/ and alcohol wipes. The forced cheer of your lobby. . . ./ I hate your winding hallways, signs pointing/ places I don't want to go."

The unwell body becomes a metaphor for marriage and marriage a metaphor for the unwell body. In her magnificent poem, "Without Our Noticing or Being Much to Blame," Shipers uses the removal of a kidney to consider the ways in which relationships can be cut too sharply for healing:

> Before his kidney was removed, my husband
> asked what would happen to the space
> where it had been. The doctor said
> his other organs would shift to fill the void.
> He promised we could lead a normal life.

But normality is impossible after a long stay in the country of illness. Shipers's unflinching poems reveal the caretaker's anger, how she is burdened by her own fidelity, the duty not to abandon a spouse in his sickness. In "Intensive Care," she confesses, "I could love/ my husband but distrust his body,/ expect betrayal at every turn." In "The Grudge I Can't Recover From," she shows a wife's loneliness transformed into rage. "I was alone when you/ were sick, and I'm alone when I remember it." Some feelings are wounds that don't heal.

If there is any hope, it is in the sequence of dog poems placed carefully throughout the collection. For Shipers, as for so many of us, the dog is both mystery and clear symbol of fidelity. In one poem, the speaker's dog, Sandbag, lives up to the many definitions of his name; he's fortification, weapon, support, a ballast. Elsewhere, the dog is a figure of grace, a creature that says *yes*—with every tail-wag, each nose-sniff—to the possibility of abundance in the world.

What *Cause for Concern* teaches us is that there are many ways a marriage can be hurt, not just through the old arguments about money, through an affair, through separate faiths or politics, but also as a result of some disaster no one could predict. Here, it is the body's betrayal, which infects the union. These are naked, open poems. They say things that make us wince, as when we look at an incision still puckered and red. "*You write/ like you're doing surgery,*" a colleague tells the speaker in the final poem of the book. And it's true. Shipers uses words as sharp scalpels, cutting away dead skin, irrigating the bleeding parts, because perhaps this is the only way to prevent infection. We can only leave the country known as illness, taking our marriages with us, when we are fully well again.

—Jehanne Dubrow

Contents

Two

Three

Cause for Concern

One

Wound Assessment

Like Thomas, the Apostle who trembles
in Caravaggio's dark light, I'm often plagued
by doubt. Twice a day, my husband sat shirtless
on a wooden chair while I pressed gauze
into his wound. The first week, I clipped my nails
so short they stung and used bare fingers.
Then I made myself wear gloves, tamp the gauze
with a sterile swab. In some paintings,
the spear wound in Christ's side emits a light
so strong the Apostles shield their eyes.
Because I only have two hands, my husband
had to hold the tape, reach for the scissors
when I was done. If he flinched or caught his breath,
I'd say, in apology and defense, *I'm doing
the best I can.* I came to hate our dining room,
stopped using the table except for mail and keys.
Sometimes I hated my husband's body,
its refusal to heal, the blood and fluid it leaked
all over the house. I hated how hard it was
to interest him in anything outside his sickness,
hated knowing we'll never escape what
we've been through. Even if we fall out of love,
divorce and never speak again, we'll still know
each other's wounds—his on the left
like Christ's, mine invisible and aching.

Carry

To transport, convey while bearing up.
Books, boxes, groceries, my dog when his feet
get cold. Purse, backpack, shopping bags,
my arms overloaded, weight bowing
my shoulders, straining my neck. At night
my knees and hipbones ache. *To bear*
or take a letter, message. My family waits
to share bad news till there's no other choice.
Giving good news discomfits me. I anticipate
objections, flaws or problems I can't see.
Champagne bubbles on my tongue but burns
my throat. *Of sound: to travel or be heard*
at a distance. Across water, wind, a room
or street, my voice loudest when least wanted,
other times too quiet, unfit to say what I
most mean. *To bear any ornament, name*
or other distinction. Some unexciting scars,
a family mole, tendency toward sarcasm
and various cancers. *To have or keep in mind.*
Stories, warnings, fears, what *could* happen
if I relax my vigilance, worries too weird
to admit except when pressed, some funny
once spoken aloud, some always frightening
no matter how unlikely. *To carry on:*
to continue, maintain, keep up or manage.
My wisest friend says *No way out but through.*
I load my bag and square my shoulders, bear

with what I can't put down, how often I
take on too much, keep what I should discard.

The History of Dogs

After Dorianne Laux

Canus lupus familiaris, descended
from the gray wolf. Predators
& scavengers, pack hunters
with complex body language,
fused wristbones & tearing teeth.
Man's best friend. Bred to hunt
& herd, stand guard & carry burdens.
Crucified in ancient Rome,
slaughtered in Malta, flayed alive
in London to show how our blood
flows. Conditioned by Pavlov
to drool on cue, sent into space,
blinded for research & better cosmetics.
The only animal that can follow
finger-points, read human faces.
Curled on our laps, against our feet,
in the center of our beds. Offered
organic food, spas & cemeteries
all their own. Driven by hunger, will eat
human remains, even of those they love.

Prayer to Our Lady of Waiting Rooms

Let the seats be plentiful and padded.
Let the magazines be recent or let the book
I've brought last until we can leave.
Let the TV on its bolted stand be off,
muted, or showing something I can ignore—
weather, game shows, CNN. Let the room
be mostly empty—no one shouting, sobbing,
asking about my husband's health.
Let everyone be strangers except
the staff. Let the walls be freshly painted,
soothing to behold. Let my husband
be there for a physical or routine checkup.
Let no one comment on my clothes
or unwashed hair, how I can sit
so calmly while he has staples
or a catheter removed, his lungs or heart
or kidneys tested, an infected wound
debrided. Under no circumstances
let me be called into the back by a nurse
who touches my arm, says *I'm sorry but*—.
Let my husband walk out whistling
before I've finished my book, looked
at my watch too many times. Let the news
be good or benign, his next appointment
not for months. When the waiting is over,
let us walk outside feeling better,
or at least no worse, than we did before.

The Absence of Trees

It was summer when we lost the trees—
overnight and all at once.
Without their deep green shade,
we liked our houses less.
The wind was warm and full of dust.
We bought more blinds and curtains,
learned to keep them closed. Without
the color and crunch of leaves,
we weren't sure when the season
changed. We found that we missed raking,
missed the smell of autumn burning
block by block. That winter,
our Christmas trees were fake and snow
fell faster than we'd ever seen.
Already our children were forgetting
tree houses and tire swings,
art they'd made with leaves
and melted wax. When we tried
to teach them about trees, we realized
how little we knew—maple, oak,
Dutch elm disease, something about moss
and being lost. We tried to describe
the shape of fruit and branches,
scrape of bark against our skin.
In our houses, what looked like wood
was usually veneer. *It's not the same,*
we said, *the trees were real.* Our children
didn't know how great our loss had been,
how much of it had been our fault.

Anti-Anxiety Poem

After Dorianne Laux

Don't worry. And when someone says *Don't worry,*
don't wonder if you're worrying enough and about
the right things. Don't worry that your headache
is really brain cancer and you'll look terrible
without your hair. When your flight is canceled
or delayed, don't assume that you aren't meant
to travel, that where you are is where you'll have
to stay. Don't double- and triple-check your purse,
fingers feeling for your wallet as nimbly
as a pickpocket's. Don't worry about pickpockets,
their dying art.

                           When the dog shits
in the dining room, don't worry he'll do it again
tomorrow and every day thereafter because
you haven't loved or walked him enough.
Don't worry about being late when you know
you're early or wear your watch on long walks
meant to clear your head. When someone asks,
What's the worst thing that could happen?
don't answer tsunami, your U-Haul stolen
and set on fire, your husband filing for divorce
for reasons you can't imagine but would probably
understand.

11

Don't worry that you've left
your doors unlocked, the oven or coffeepot on.
Don't worry that running out of concrete fears—
a flat tire, bad test results, suspicious charge
to your account—will leave you open to the vague
and nameless dread you'd do anything to avoid.
Don't try to explain, even to those you love,
the dilemmas you've faced by 9 a.m., the deathbeds
you've visited, disasters you've seen or averted.
Don't worry that worry might be all you have.

How Sandbag Lives Up to His Name

As fortification: I'd never have a child
to save my marriage but thought a dog
might help—something we could love
that wouldn't talk, hold our human flaws
against us as we often do each other's.
Something to focus on besides our work,
my husband's health. *As a weapon:*
I worry about his weight, his walks, how long
his nails should be. His seizures worry
both of us but I'm the one who counts
his pills, calls the vet, records date, duration
and severity. *As support:* He doesn't like
for me to cry, slide on ice, get dizzy
and have to sit down. When my husband
stays home sick, sometimes I'm jealous
of their naps, how much they watch TV.
To exclude a draft: I can't imagine how
I lived without his warm weight on my lap,
wedged against hip or spine when I sleep.
Even in winter I wake up sweating.
Other nights I'm cold, pat the blankets to find
he's scooted away from me or gotten up
when my husband did. *As ballast:*
If he holds us down, keeps us from going out
or sleeping in, he makes sure we don't
float away from each other, the life
we've made but sometimes want to escape.

Migration

If gulls are the souls of drowned sailors,
I understand why they choose Nebraska,
the Hy-Vee parking lot where they dive
and cry while I load groceries into my trunk.
In November, my husband almost drowned
in his own body. The day he was moved
to the ICU, I bought jeans and cardigans,
lotion I didn't need. It was nearly Christmas,
and no one in those bright stores knew
my husband wasn't well and hadn't been
for months, that my hair was falling out
in handfuls, that I wanted to fly away
and not come home till he was healed,
our lives wiped clean of blood and worry.
Instead, I pushed gauze into his wound,
laundry into machines, a grocery cart
down shining aisles where everything
was without damage or history.

My husband didn't drown. He came home
in a week, was back at work within a month.
My hair grew thick again, my laugh
less bitter. I found other things to think about
besides his health, my own fatigue.
I thought about the gulls, the wind that led them
so far from the sea, whether they cried—
if they cried, instead of called or screamed—
for the ocean, everything they'd lost.

Letter from a Place I've Just Arrived

It's lovely here, the leaves just starting
to turn, but at night I hear strange noises
coming from the hills. I'm told wild dogs
have colonized the dump. Other sounds

are more like screams—coyotes, maybe,
or the feral cats that pile moles and robins
beside my door. People aren't as friendly
as they seem. They smile and ask how I am

but refuse to meet for lunch or coffee.
Even the mums I bought were a mistake.
My neighbor said since she has gold,
I need orange. When I mentioned it

to the mail carrier, he took my neighbor's side.
Also, he said it was too early to put out
pumpkins, even if they weren't carved.
I tried going to the library, but the books

I need are ruined, half the pages missing,
others marked with thick black ink.
I don't mean to complain so much.
I'm told the apples are amazing,

that I'll love my first snow. But sometimes
the howling makes it hard to sleep,
and it gets dark a little sooner every day.
By afternoon, my hands are stiff and cold.

Fidelis

*Because watchdogs failed to warn Rome of the attacking Gauls
in 380 BC, each year dogs were ritually crucified near the
temple of Juventas.*

They know when they've been chosen. They cower
and cry, lick or bite the hands that grab their scruffs
and drag them to the cross. Mostly we take strays,

though we always need a pet or two—clean, collared,
well-fed—to show that justice rules us all. Their paws,
held still for nail and mallet, smell like grass, like dew

and rising bread. If the watchdogs had done their job,
signaled *stranger* and *attack,* we'd be spared our task,
pity we feel but have to hide. Men may scream or faint,

but most await their deaths with glazed acceptance.
Unless we crack their skulls or cut their throats to make
them quiet, dogs howl and whimper to the end. What must

they think of us, their source of food and shelter turned
to beasts more vicious than themselves? Is knowledge
of the watchdogs' failure, bodies on the cross, passed

from bitch to pup, within a pack or household? We know
what dogs deserve, but not how much they understand
of sin, punishment, payment for betrayal.

Confession

When you aren't sure what to write about, write about something you can't tell your mother.
—James Allen Hall

I stopped calling because you didn't
always seem glad to hear from me.
Last week, my dog got more medical care
than I did during my entire childhood,
and he wasn't even sick. I don't talk
to my brother because he's an angry drunk.
When I was a teenager, I lied a lot
more often than I got caught. I hardly ever
wash my sheets or save the greeting cards
you send for Halloween or Groundhog Day.
Your coffee makes my stomach hurt.
I have friends whose advice I actually follow.
I can never tell that you've lost weight,
don't always trust you'll take my side.
When you say you're worried about me,
I feel like I've done something wrong.
I knew I was moving to Wisconsin
for months before I told you. Because
I'll never be ready to live without you,
I have to practice while you're still alive.

Dear Hospital,

I hate your smell of potatoes
and alcohol wipes. The forced cheer of your lobby,
with its dried flowers and holiday displays.
Your elderly volunteers, their kindly greetings
and inability to answer any question except
where the restrooms are. I hate your coffee shop,
its weak brew and insufficient hours,
live piano music that sets my teeth on edge.
I hate your winding hallways, signs pointing
places I don't want to go. Your waiting rooms,
awkwardly arranged and stocked with pamphlets—
*What to Expect in the ICU, When Caregivers
Give Too Much*—I shove in my purse
when no one's looking. I even hate your chapel,
which is too close to the elevators although at least
it's dimly lit. The plastic shoes your nurses wear.
Your parking garage, the NO SMOKING policy
that covers your entire campus. I hate
that you call it a *campus*. Dear Hospital,
I hate how many of your windows
I've looked through, how many hours I've spent
observing your routines. I hate how safe
you make me feel, how every time
we leave I worry it's too soon.

John Wayne

After Dorianne Laux

I've never understood how I should feel
about John Wayne—an American hero
who never went to war, was racist, sexist,
imperialist, and loud. But when I watch
his movies, I fall for it all—the swagger
and drawl, shoot-from-the-hip, hat pulled low,
the hint (and sometimes more than hint)
of violence in his kiss, his big hands gripping
the face or shoulders of the female lead,
some too young for him by decades, but who
turns down John Wayne? Not his three wives,
women he cheated with and on, studio heads
who let him make disasters like *The Conqueror.*
I try to forget his later films, *The Cowboys,*
The Shootist, the West disappearing on film
as it did in life, John disappearing
into stomach cancer and caricature, into legend
though he was still alive. *The Searchers*
might be his best work but it's not my favorite.
I like *McClintock!, Big Jake,* and god
forgive me, *Hatari!,* an endorsement of zoos
and manifest destiny but hilarious if I don't
think too hard. I know he had regrets—
choosing movies over war in 1941,
playing Davy Crockett just to get *The Alamo*

made—but in *She Wore a Yellow Ribbon,*
he calls apology a sign of weakness. Like all
his fans, I take what I want from him
and leave the rest behind. Because I have
so many doubts, I need him to have none.

Self-Portrait as Dog

Sometimes I bark because I'm scared
I don't exist. Sometimes I listen
with my whole body hoping
for your approach. I snap because
my jaws were made to bite,
close my teeth around your wrist
or hem because I need your fingers
in my fur, need you to see the belly
I trust you won't rip out. Even
when it looks like I'm asleep
I'm watching you for clues:
How close may I sit? How long
will you stay? How much
of what you're eating may I have?
I know I have terrible breath,
a problem with boundaries. I have
to shove my snout into your armpit,
crotch, ear, memorize your smell
in case you're ever lost. In the dreams
I can't describe, I don't chase
cats or rabbits, I chase you.
I need you to love me all the time,
even when I'm least deserving.

He Watches the Weather Channel

After Reagan Lothes

Because nothing else is on so early
in the morning when he drinks coffee
in an empty house. Because almanacs

are of limited use compared to satellites.
Because spring will have to come somehow
and cold reminds him which bones

he's broken. Because every flight delayed
or canceled is one he won't be on. Because
people should stay where they're from,

except his children, who were right to leave.
Because a flood will take what it can
and move uphill. Because just once

he'd like to see a tornado touch down
in an empty field and go away
hungry. Because his wife nearly died

on an icy road. Because he can't prepare
for disasters he doesn't understand.
Because wind keeps him awake. Because

his boots are by the door but his slicker
is in his truck. Because he can't change
a damn thing forecast and uncertainty aches

like a tired muscle, an unhealed wound.

The Memorial Circus

Inspired by a mishearing of "memorial service"

                                        was well-attended.
Only a close observer could've seen
what was amiss: the ringmaster wore
his usual tails but left his mustache
unwaxed, his top hat slightly askew.
The lion hardly roared, his shaggy head
too heavy for his rumpled neck,
and the elephants couldn't keep time.
The knife-thrower's aim was off,
his assistant petrified. The jugglers
dropped nothing but lacked
their usual flair, plucking clubs
and torches from the air by rote.
Mid-lift, the strongman froze
and shook until the clowns appeared,
their greasepaint faces firmly drawn.
Twice, the trapeze swung empty
when aerialists missed their tricks;
the wire-walkers bobbled but stayed
aloft. Only the illusionist seemed
untouched, his doves and rabbits
appearing right on cue, but the lilies
he produced were past their prime.

Afterward, the audience stomped
and clapped and whistled while performers
bowed and waved, wished they'd all
go home. Backstage, the rousties' backs
and shoulders throbbed. It would take
all night to pack up props, break down
bleachers and collapse tents, right
every twisted rope and tangled winch.
But even they had to admit: the memorial
circus was a great success. The crowd
had no idea what they'd just seen.

When you embark on a catastrophe,

no matter how carefully you chart your course,
you'll be lost as soon as the shore recedes.
Alone in the captain's quarters, you'll drop
the sextant and muddle the compass. What you see
of stars will only add to your confusion.
You'll stand watch until you're dazed with boredom,
drop into your hammock and wake to the worst
of a storm, lightning striking the mast,
the rigging tangled, sails torn. As soon as you
batten the hatches, the sun will appear.

You'll find yourself becalmed, with too much
ballast and not enough wind. Salt will split
your lips and sting your skin. Hungry
for horizon, you'll think you've sighted land
so often you'll stop believing the spyglass,
your own excited cries. Your crew will look
to you for answers and find that you have none.
They'll be surly and often drunk, but you'll
fear mutiny too much to have them flogged.
The only ships you'll see will be flying
enemy flags, too far for you to hail.

You'll hear rumors of an island to the east
and consider rowing there, armed only
with an ax and a bag of biscuits. You'll find
the lifeboat only has one oar, that its stores

were raided weeks ago. Besides, you'll know
you're supposed to go down with the ship,
even when the wreck isn't your fault.

Undone

Let's face it. We're undone by each other. And if we're not,
we're missing something. If this seems so clearly the case
with grief, it is only because it was already the case with
desire. One does not always stay intact.

　　　—Judith Butler

I wanted to bring his kidney home in a jar,
keep it on the mantel or shelf above our bed
like a souvenir, proof of what we survived.
Sometimes I want my husband to lift his shirt
and show his scar—the eighteen-inch incision
like a magician's trick gone wrong, the mouth-
shaped groove left by infection we fought
for two months straight. I want someone
to ask what it was like: the surgery itself,
which took more time and blood than planned.
The night we called the fire department
because he couldn't get off the couch. How nice
they were, how I hated for them to leave.
The abscess. Pneumonia. The oxygen tank
in our bedroom. The sleep study, blood clots,
shots that bruised his belly. His bad moods
and helplessness. My hair falling out,
my world reduced to a series of waiting rooms
and British mysteries I kept in my purse.
There's so much my husband has forgotten
or never knew: how angry I was and how

much grief I felt, how I carried his sickness
everywhere I went. How he'll never
make it up to me, settle this debt I'm ashamed
to admit exists. How I can't imagine
our marriage without this disaster in it.

Two

Voice of God

I know *dog* is *god* spelled backward
but not what my dog believes,
what he sees when his brain short-circuits
into seizures that make his eyes roll
and back legs tremble. Last November,
I heard the voice of God. He said,
Get out of Nebraska, you stupid slut.
He said, *Don't pretend I don't exist.*
If I were a woman with a small child,
would you stop for me then? God
was wearing a flannel shirt, jeans dark
with dirt, and drinking from a bottle of—
let's call it rye or bourbon, not vodka
or champagne. I was wearing
a leather coat and walking a dachshund
on a leash longer than I am tall.

Because we like to walk fast and without
interruption, we were a block away
when God shouted, *People don't know*
what they don't know. I looked over
my shoulder: he stood with arms
outstretched, bottle in his fist. I unlocked
our door, fed the dog his dinner, a pill
hidden in a piece of cheese. I tried
to understand what the message meant.

Intensive Care

The night I was summoned to the ICU,
I took a toothbrush, contact solution
and extra socks. I changed my sweater
so I'd smell less like smoke, the greasy meal
that made my stomach hurt.
My husband's room had sliding glass doors
and an intubation kit on the counter.
I told them to call in the morning, he said,
voice muffled by the oxygen mask.
I stayed for exactly fifteen minutes
before picking up my heavy bag. I'd come
prepared for an emergency, and since
there wasn't one, I wanted to go home.

When I say, *the year my husband almost died,*
I mean how it felt, the mixture of urgency
and exhaustion that settled in my bones
and brain, affected everything I did,
but I never really thought that he might die.
Every day he was home felt like a test—
of patience, endurance, how much
I loved him and wanted him well.
When he was in the hospital,
I often felt relief: he was surrounded
by people who knew what to do.

I didn't know *well* was a relative term,
that we'd never get back the life we had
before his sickness, that I could love
my husband but distrust his body,
expect betrayal at every turn.

The Rapture

Using mathematical evidence from the Bible, Christian radio host Harold Camping predicted the Rapture would occur on May 21, 2011.

Last Saturday the Rapture failed to come.
I assumed that I'd be left behind
but all day wondered how I'd act
if I believed: Would I still clean my house?
Buy frozen food? Pay my rent? To live
expecting Armageddon's day and hour
takes a kind of faith I've never had.
People left their jobs, let the bank
foreclose and worked twelve-hour days
to spread the word, give the rest of us
one more last chance. I can't imagine
how they felt as the appointed hour passed,
then another, a day, a string of them.
What do they think of the world
they're still in—reporters anxious
to embarrass them, bank accounts run dry,
milk and licenses they've let expire?
That Sunday morning could've been
the best or worst they'd ever seen—
irises in bloom, highway signs for churches
and cheap gas, plastic pennants rattling
the breeze. Nothing here's as perfect
as the Heaven they were trusting in,

but I hope they see how hard
the rest of us are trying, how we find
redemption everywhere we can.

The Dogs of Malta, 1565

At first they were easy to kill: we called,
they came, laid heads on knees or stood
with paws against our chests. We slit
their throats, opened velvet bellies and used
their guts to poison wells. We killed
hunters and herders, lapdogs who'd slept
beside our beds or in them. Most died
without protesting, but some smelled blood
on our hands, murder in our hearts.
Surrounded by the sea, packs ran
from shore to shore unable to escape.

At the siege of Rhodes, people grew so hungry
they ate dogs that fed on human corpses.
To save both us and them from such disgrace,
boys aged ten to twelve were given knives,
a bounty for each kill. The Turkish horde
sails closer every day while dogs grow fewer
and more fierce. Three boys have died already,
brought down by curs that once were trusted pets.

Heaps of skin and bone rot faster than they burn.
Our women safe in other places, we live
on an island of men and dogs. Like us,
our enemies will find one set of howling jaws
and bloody teeth is much like another,
though we move upright and with less grace.

"Suppose, suppose—"

Wyatt Earp's last words, January 13, 1929

Suppose his first wife hadn't died
so soon after their wedding,
that he hadn't spent the next eleven years
in and running from disgrace,
hunting buffalo and working in bordellos.
Suppose he'd had better luck
at cards and politics, that all men
kept their word as well as he did.
Suppose his neck had been less stiff,
his hips less lean and saddle-ready.
Suppose he hadn't been a handsome man,
never loved Doc Holliday or left Dodge.
Suppose he'd died in the Tombstone
shoot-out he helped start and hadn't seen,
in the weeks that followed, two brothers
shot from ambush, one crippled
and one killed. Suppose he'd been
arrested, tried and hanged for the men
he killed on his Vendetta Ride.
Suppose headlines and poverty
hadn't haunted his old age. Suppose
he'd died of lead poisoning instead
of cystitis or lived to see and profit from
the myth his life became. Suppose
even half the stories told were true.

My Life in the Circus

Shovel, pitchfork, hose. Hay stuck to my shirt,
ears shut against the braying calls: *I'm hungry*
I'm hungry I miss my home. The elephants
have names I never use, though I've learned
to read their rolling eyes and restless feet
for signs of boredom or fatigue. They don't think
of me at all beyond the food I bring, water
washing gray-brown backs, salve I smear
inside their irons.

          Most days the work's
no worse than on my father's farm, even with
the hissing cats, music turned flat and tinny
by speakers I hate to rig. Folks here
don't ask each other questions. We do
our jobs, put on our show, then tear it down
and disappear. When people complain it's not
what they expected—everything a little tattered,
torn and then repaired—they mean it's like
the world they know.

          Before I came,
the oldest cow pulled up her stakes,
tossed her handler and a couple clowns
and headed for the highway, where a rifle
ended her escape. The others aren't disturbed
by storms, mice I throw into their stalls,

but if I shorted their food, struck the hook
against their slender trunks, tightened
their shackles until they rubbed—
imagine all that animal rage and grief aimed,
for once, at its right target, people and what
we've done, a reckoning as fierce as we deserve.

Without Our Noticing or Being Much to Blame

Because kidneys are easier to add
than subtract, some transplant recipients
have as many as five inside their bodies.
Some websites match people who need
a kidney with strangers willing to donate one,
an act that's either heroic or bizarre.
Unlike heart or brain or spleen,
kidneys lack metaphorical uses—
they don't break or burn, get blamed
for bad decisions. The only myth
about them I know is an urban legend—
Mexico or Vegas, the hotel bathtub
filled with ice, the groggy patient
fingering his stitches. One working kidney
is enough, though twice my husband's
has been described as lazy and threatened
with temporary dialysis. The more I learn
about our bodies the more mysterious
they seem, full of pockets and alcoves
where things go wrong without
our noticing or being much to blame.
Before his kidney was removed, my husband
asked what would happen to the space
where it had been. The doctor said
his other organs would shift to fill the void.
He promised we could lead a normal life.

At the Sadness Factory,

                                    every shift
is overnight or double. Always, layoffs
loom. When the lunch bell rings,
the line creaks to a halt and workers eat
dry sandwiches brought from home,
bruised fruit, leftovers in the fridge too long.
They have to swallow hard to overcome
their knotted throats. Talk of weather
or local sports can lead to tears.
The suggestion box is empty and quotas
go unmet. As the market shrank,
other plants diversified or just
shut down. Now most of their products
go overseas on cargo boats that sink
or simply vanish. Old-timers say
they used to work harder but for better pay.
They look forward to retirement,
small pensions and trips to the lake,
though they'll miss the hum and bustle,
the birthdays marked with cake and used
balloons, bowling and softball teams
that lose or have to forfeit. Supervisors
are sadder than folks on the line,
the managers saddest of all. The owner
used to be sad but now comes only
at Christmas, bringing whiskey
no one drinks. The Sadness Factory is,
as it's always been, the town's largest
employer. No one believes it could close.

Love Poem to a Murder Ballad

We'll meet behind the barn, beside the river,
high on the mountain by my father's house
on a night the moon is bright and full. Liquor
on your breath, devil in your eyes, you want

to marry me, lay me in the grass or deny
what we've already done. I know you've come
to kill me, lover. Lips stinging from my kiss,
you'll stab me in the back I've turned, shoot me

through my milk-white breast, smash my skull
against a stone. When the chorus comes,
you'll say you didn't know our love
was leading here, wept when you saw

what you'd done. Or else felt no remorse at all,
scrubbed blood from hands and shirt and rode
your horse to town. No matter how you hide
my body, the evidence all points to you. You know

the tree from which you'll hang, white oak
or locust, branches waiting for the rope.
I might become a ghost, uneasy in my grave,
haunting you if your heart doesn't. I might

become a tale to frighten girls into staying home
and having no desires, the song men hear
when they've done wrong. Murder ballad, you mean
me harm from your first note but I still sing along.

Home Health

When you live inside *emergency,*
you may leave for work an hour early,
wish you could stay late. In the hospital,
someone else prepares the food, does dishes
and laundry, decides when to call for aid.
At home, you do all these things
at once or do nothing but talk yourself
into taking a shower, putting on shoes
and mascara before making your escape.
In the grocery checkout line you feel
exposed, sure your cart will give you away—
7-UP, yogurt, soup. If anyone asks
how you are, you won't tell the truth—
angry, tired, sad, uncertain, tired again.

Your friends suggest that you get help,
but no one offers what you need—
a fairy godmother who's also a registered nurse,
whose comfort you'd believe. You want
your husband healed, though you'd settle
for more present and in less pain,
want to close the door and lock
what hurts you out instead of in.

In your next letter,

please describe
the weather in great detail. If possible,
enclose a fist of snow or mud,

everything you know about the soil,
how tomato leaves rub green against
your skin and make you itch, how slow

the corn is growing on the hill.
Thank you for the photographs
of where the chicken coop once stood,

clouds that did not become tornadoes.
When I try to explain where I'm from,
people imagine corn bread, cast-iron,

cows drifting across grass. I interrupt
with barbed wire, wind, harvest air
that reeks of wheat and diesel.

I hope your sleep comes easy now
that you've surrendered the upstairs,
hope the sun still lets you drink

one bitter cup before its rise. I don't miss
flannel shirts, radios with only
AM stations, but there's a certain kind

of star I can't see from where I am—
bright, clear, unconcerned. I need
your recipes for gravy, pie crust,

canned green beans. I'm sending you
the buttons I can't sew back on.
Please put them in the jar beside your bed.

In your next letter, please send seeds
and feathers, a piece of bone or china
you plowed up last spring. Please

promise I'm missing the right things.

The Notion of Dog

I worry about my dignity and Dog says *yes*
to licking paws and penis, scratching an itch
because he can, *yes* to peeing on piles of leaves,
the neighbors' tomato plants, sidewalk
when it snows. I worry about my weight
and Dog says *yes* to food he finds
in the grass, pizza crusts and chicken wings,
donuts with one bite gone. I worry
about causing scenes and Dog says *yes*
to sniffing strangers' feet, barking at dogs
he doesn't know, yanking his leash
toward what he needs to see. I worry
about working hard enough and Dog
says *yes* to chasing birds he'll never catch,
yes to napping in the afternoon, herding me
toward bed because he's tired. Because Dog
says *yes* he brings me grace, a world
where abundance is expected and received.

Self-Portrait as Donald Crowhurst

While competing in an around-the-world yacht race in 1969, Crowhurst began reporting false coordinates while stalled in the Atlantic Ocean. Eleven days after his last radio transmission, his boat was found unoccupied and adrift.

If this boat were an island, if stars would just hold still
If wind would fill my sails

If I could trust the log I wrote with my own hand
If I'd had more time to prepare, pack supplies I knew I'd need

If piracy seemed possible
If I could sail my boat as well as it deserves

If the ocean were less itself and more as I imagined it
If my lips weren't made of salt

If the clock would stop its ticking
If I remembered which lies I've told the radio, which I've written down

If a whale would swallow me and spit me out on shore
If my return might go unnoticed

If the others would arrive at where they think I am
If I could choose my end

Wind Rattling the Stalks

A Massachusetts family got the Halloween scare of a lifetime by getting lost inside a dark and creepy Salem-area corn maze and had to call 911 for rescue.

—msnbc.com, 10/12/2011

My first call was treated like a prank.
Good luck with that, the woman said.
But my baby was brand-new and it
was getting dark. We had one small blanket,
my thin sweater, no way to survive
the night. We heard trucks on the highway,
wind rattling the stalks. I told myself
I wouldn't cry, that I'd be like the women
who lifted cars off injured children,
fought bears and tigers with bare hands,
ran into burning houses to find their babies.
My husband's knees and back were sore.
If I had to leave him behind, I'd fold
the blanket into a sling for the baby,
take my toddler by the hand. I'd walk
till we were home. I called for help again,
tried to sound calm, polite, like someone
police would want to save. Finally—
sirens, search dogs, an officer who swept
my son into his arms. Outside the maze,
more police, reporters, the owner offering

pumpkins and cups of cider, saying
at least no one was harmed. Later, people
would laugh, *Only lost for ninety minutes.*
Called 911 and *twenty-five feet from the exit.*
When I became a mother, I swore
I'd give anything to keep my children safe.
My dignity was easy to surrender.

The Grudge I Can't Recover From

After Elizabeth Wade

You weren't there when I sat in the waiting room,
book on my lap, earphones in, trying not
to wonder what your chances were.
You weren't there when I went home
and stuffed myself with grease and ice cream
that made my stomach ache or when I dreamed
of ringing phones, hospital hallways with signs
I couldn't read. Even after you came home,
you weren't really there when I washed
bloody laundry, made scrambled eggs
and endless trips to the pharmacy, or when I slept
or cried in the ten-minute lulls between
your calls. You were looking the other way
when I rolled my eyes, stuck out my tongue
or mouthed *Shut up* because I couldn't fix
a single thing that made you hurt. You weren't there
when I thought about escape, staying
on the interstate long past the exit home.
Are you mad at me? you ask on days I snap
or sigh and shake my head in your direction.
What did I do wrong? I can't admit the grudge
I can't recover from: I was alone when you
were sick, and I'm alone when I remember it.

Killing the Messenger

Our god took a tenth of every harvest,
our fattest sheep and finest cloth. On holy days
we cut our hair, smeared ourselves with ash
or opened veins and offered him our blood.
But we also sang, played drums and cymbals,
danced to celebrate the seasons, marriages
and births. Because our god lived far away,
was hard to look upon, we chose a go-between
to speak with him and bring back word.

He said our god was displeased by dancing,
that we should destroy our harps and drums,
keep our voices plain and low. Then singing,
too, was disallowed. Our god still let us
gather and quietly rejoice, but we grew weary
as his demands increased—more sheep
and grain, more wine and woven cloth.
We sent our go-between to tell
our god how hard we had to work,
how much we missed music and dance.

He said our god had threatened plague,
threatened to smite us all and start again
with followers who had more faith.
We wondered why our god had grown
so angry, made our go-between repeat
his words until his voice was cracked

and broken. We decided hunger would change
his mind, and if not hunger, perhaps thirst,
bruises left by stones we threw.
Once he was dead, we began to sing, to dance
and play the instruments we'd hidden.
We knew he'd lied, knew our god
would smile on what we'd done. Our next
go-between would need to serve us better.

Argos

In Homer's The Odyssey *(Book 17), when Odysseus returned to Ithaca in disguise after twenty years' absence, only his dog recognized him. Argos died after his master walked past him into the palace.*

They say I waited because loyalty is in my nature,
because I could only love Odysseus, who bred me
for the hunt but left before I was weaned. Other men
made use of me: my legs were strong and liked

to cover ground. I outran deer and wild goats,
flushed rabbits toward the bows. Men praised
my nose and scratched my flanks, but none
would take me home, let me lie against his feet

and guard his children. Then came the hunt
I couldn't lead, paws stalled as if in mud
but on dry ground. One day I heard men gather
in the yard and limped outside, bones sore but willing.

Shut inside the stable, I had too much pride to howl—
my hunting days were done because men said
they were. Boys brought bits of meat but didn't
come too close. My fur was rank and full of fleas,

jaws prone to snap. They say I stayed alive
to see him one last time, that I alone knew
he'd return. The truth is that my heart kept beating,
legs dragging me toward sun. I heard his voice,

heard his companion speak my name. Too weak
to rise, I wagged my tail, watched them both walk on.
All the time they thought I waited for Odysseus,
I would've served any man who wanted me.

After the Piper

There was no more school, no more games
on the village green. There was only me
and a handful of babies too young to crawl.
My father wanted to send me away,
but the priest said no, the village had need
of a child. Some women wept
and gave me sweets. Men pressed pennies
into my palms, said I was growing strong.
Other parents ran indoors when they saw me
or ignored me altogether. I thought I'd leave
when I got older, not knowing as soon
as I said my name—not even Hamelin,
just my name—and stepped with my limping leg,
everyone would know where I was from.

In church, a window stained my face
with colored light—rats, piper, children, road.
Tragedies, says the priest, are also acts of God.
No one knows what made the window fall—
a heavy wind, misguided bird, someone
throwing stones. The pieces were smashed
too fine to fix, leading scattered in the grass.
Would I have followed the piper
if I could? Even if it meant the mountain,
rock closing over me, no way to come home?
No one saw: my survival was also a sacrifice.

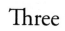

Three

When He'll Be Well and Stay That Way

Five days after we move to Wisconsin
I'm sitting in a hospital parking lot
while my husband has three stitches removed
from his left hand. His injury—a lesion
in his palm that bled and had to be repaired—
isn't serious, and for once I didn't learn
the condition's name or usual causes.
I want to know when he'll be well
and stay that way, when his body will stop
failing us both, an unfair question I ask
every time we're here again, *here* meaning
any hospital, doctor's office or specialty clinic.
I'd feel better if he were to blame for all
the ways he's been unwell since we
got married, but it's probably genetics
or just bad luck. *I didn't sign up for this,*
I sometimes think, as though anyone does,
as though I couldn't be hit by a car
tomorrow and shift the burden onto him.
I'm terrified by things I can't control
and ignore them when I can. His health
feels like a hurricane inside our house,
like punishment for sins I don't remember.
To protect myself, I track his appointments,
nag about exercise and medication.
He can't keep himself from getting sick
any more than I can make or keep him well,
but sometimes I wish he'd try harder.

If Dogs Could Talk

If dogs could talk they might recall their puppyhood,
their mother's tongue, shock of light when their eyes
first opened, the loneliness of leaving home.
Perhaps they'd lie about squirrels they've bagged,

hands they've bitten, escapes they've made,
or brag about their bodies, their strong legs
and sturdy chests, the keenness of their hearing.
Maybe they'd compare their neighborhoods, where

to find bread meant for birds, bones with chicken
still attached, pools of grease to coat their tongues.
Maybe they'd console each other about the vet,
sting of shots that treats can't ease. Or recount

the dreams that make their tails and noses twitch,
hazy, half-remembered scenes of running in a pack,
of hunting or herding, doing their jobs well.
If we appeared at all it might be in complaints—

how short their walks, how long they wait
for our return. How we jerk the leash, forget
to fill their bowls and give too many baths.
Our clumsy feet, obsession with where they piss

and shit. If dogs could talk we might discover
we don't know how they think or what they value,
that our lives are parallel but not entwined, that we
don't have a starring role in what they'd say.

Heaven

After Mark Doty

It's easy to accessorize the afterlife:
let there be corn bread for R.,
a shaded riverbank where he can fish.
A. needs open water, sailboats and kayaks,
fruit always in season. For me, books
and country songs, a dog to walk—
as if Heaven is like our lives but without
the distractions of paying bills,
preparing meals we may not want.
When I fly, I always book
a window seat, always try to keep
my eyes open, fists unclenched,
as those jet engines rush us toward
the sky—but once we've leveled off,
I read, fidget with my purse, wonder
how well I've packed, what I've left
at home. When we're in Heaven,
I suppose we'll do what folks
in Heaven do and we won't worry
if it's not what we expected or regret
what we don't have. Which sounds
like acceptance, when really I mean
I may be wrong about what Heaven is
but can't stop picturing a place
that offers everything we need.

Self-Portrait as Aerialist

I've always been afraid to fall—the rough
embrace of the net, the crowd's shocked gasp,
my mother's disapproval. She loves me best

when I can fly, when I trust the bar, the leap,
the air and all my training. From far away,
every catch, release and tumble looks as effortless

as breath. Up close, we grunt and cry, hands
sweat and slip, wires creak and nearly tangle.
I'd rather be the girl the magician disappears,

the lovely target spinning for the knives,
assistant who holds the hoops the cats
jump through—anything to avoid the long climb

and quick launch into space where only light
will catch me every time. Every landing
comes as a relief, the platform trembling

beneath my feet, ache in my chest easing.
If I crash into the net I have to wave and smile,
pretend it doesn't hurt to fall so far.

Invitation to a Lingering Fall

The first frost caught me by surprise.
I didn't cover what I should have,
bring my blooms inside. Most days start
with fog, this cough that I can't shake.

I know November can't be helped,
but it's September and I'm sorry I moved
north. Already the leaves look spent,
are barely hanging on. The only place

I feel completely warm is in my car,
the heater turned on high when I drive
to the store. I crave potatoes, carrots,
beets—anything to roast and eat

with too much butter. I'm already wearing
my wool socks, sweaters I meant to save.
I'd like to know how other folks survive—
I still see people in short sleeves,

see them grilling meals they eat outside.
I'd love for you to come, even if you
can't stay. We could find out if my fireplace
works, buy cider from a roadside stand.

You could help me close up holes
where mice get in, seal cracks
before it snows. If you were here,
I might not mind when winter comes.

Love Poem to Ted Neeley in *Jesus Christ Superstar*

Lincoln, NE, 2009

That man's too old to play Christ, someone said
when you appeared onstage—thirty years
in those white robes, spotlights tracking
your graceful sleeves, the attentive angle
of your head as you worked a crowd. I agreed
that you looked tired, but when Mary Magdalene
anointed you, when you cast merchants
and money changers from the temple, I forgot
your thinning hair and wrinkled brow, forgot
how your story ended: your broken voice
crying on the cross, your body arched as you
ascended. I'd lost track of how many songs
were in the second act, thought there might
be more—the empty tomb, your appearance
on the road, to Peter in Jerusalem—but the cast
came out for applause: soldiers, Apostles,
and women; Annas, Caiaphas, Pilate; Mary
in her red dress; Peter, that sturdy fisherman;
Judas, who has all the best songs; and finally
you, head bowed at our ovation. I didn't come
to worship but you've left me no choice.
I don't care how old you are, how many times
you've done this act before—you still rock
those power ballads, still heal with the same
sweet force before you rise. Tonight, I'll believe
until the curtain closes, tour bus rolls away.

In Certain Light

I didn't know what to do with Death
after I moved. I left it in the garage
at first, then hauled it to the basement
with other things I'd brought but didn't use—
curling iron, stereo, a lamp missing
its shade. I knew I couldn't donate Death
or leave it on the curb, but I was
running out of shelves, vowed not
to clutter the counters. Doing laundry,
I listened for Death's dry cough.
I dreamed the box got wet and started
to buckle, dreamed Death climbed
the stairs, was waiting in the dining room,
beside my bed. I opened the box
to make the nightmares stop—bubble wrap,
newspaper, dish towels shoved in the corners—
and turned Death over in my hands.
The only damage was a dent from years ago
when I'd seen Death as something
I could fight or else ignore. I'd forgotten
how heavy it was, how warm against
my skin, forgotten how it shone
in certain light. I carried it upstairs,
set it on the sill above my kitchen sink.
If I had to live with Death,
I'd keep it out for everyone to see.

Something Other than a Problem to Be Solved

The closer my husband got to being well,
the further away from him I waited
when I drove him to the doctor, making
my way from exam room to waiting area
to hospital lobby. Eventually I stayed in the car,
book open on the steering wheel. He never
asked me why but I explained it anyway—
the weather was nice, he wouldn't be long,
I was saving myself the walk inside.
When he was very sick, his illness felt
like a hole I'd fallen into, weight that crushed
my chest. I had dreams about drowning
and being lost, which mostly stopped
when he got mostly well, though I still
struggle with waiting rooms, believing
he's fully healed. To protect myself
when he was sick, I learned to keep
his body, health, comfort separate
from my own. Now I worry I'm not close
enough, that if I can't think of him
as something other than a problem to be solved,
disaster waiting to happen, our marriage
won't survive what we've been through.

Trade Agreement

It's hard to know if my dog loves me
specifically or in the abstract. Evidence
suggests dogs mostly tamed themselves,

that they hung around human settlements
eating trash and warning off intruders
until we took them in. Because my dog

was four when I adopted him, he's had
other lives I don't know much about—
I don't think he was abused, can tell

he was taught to sit and walk on-leash,
only pee outdoors. But I don't know
how he felt about those other homes,

if he liked them more or less than he
likes mine. Experts claim we get more
from dogs than we can give, that,

having traded affection for food
and shelter, they've been made to suffer
misguided breeding and benign neglect,

the boredom of being alone all day.
My dog knows my smell and the sound
of my voice, pressure of my palms

against his fur. He knows his meals
and walks mostly arrive on time. If what
he feels for me is love, he can't say it

in words I'd understand for sure. If he
feels something else—fear, frustration,
gratitude—I'm happier not knowing.

Animal Control

In October 2011, the owner of an exotic animal farm near Zanesville, OH, set his animals free before taking his own life.

We mostly ticket speeders, write up car thefts
and break-ins, look for meth labs before
they blow. When the sheriff said shoot to kill
we nodded, shouldered rifles we rarely use.
I admit we did some bragging—how true
our aim had been, how those lions and bears
would snarl in surprise, then topple over
in slow motion. But once we'd cleaned
our weapons and gone home, seen the footage
of all those fierce and lovely creatures reduced
to rotting meat—none of us stayed proud
of what we'd done.

                              The animals weren't
to blame, not for how they were kept
or making us afraid. But we had to protect
our county, the school kids and soccer moms,
older folks on nearby farms. I saw the tiger
they tried to tranquilize, saw it turn and leap,
jaws snapping like the gunshots that followed.
After the owner opened all the cages, he broke
the locks. He either wanted us to shoot
on sight or hoped the animals would make it
to the woods, find some way to survive.

When I take my kids to the zoo, the big cats
all look bored and restless, lions roaring
at the highway behind their habitat.
They can't see the road but they can hear it.
They know they aren't where they belong,
that they should run if they get the chance.

What I've Learned and Would Like to Forget

He recovers slowly from anesthesia,
has trouble breathing and forming words.
He likes blankets from the warmer,
being asked about his work. He likes the food,
how it simply appears on plastic trays,
and insists on clean socks brought from home,
underwear when he can wear it.

How to pack for a hospital visit: sweater,
book, granola bars, memo pad and pen.
I get his doctors' names confused,
like his nurses less than I should.
Sitting beside his bed, I get bored, worry
I'm staying too long or leaving too soon.

When he's released, he forgets I'm not
a nurse, that I don't know his pills or how
to give them. I panic when there's no need,
dismiss what's cause for concern. He cries
from pain and frustration. I cry because I'm tired,
because sometimes I want to leave him
in the hospital lobby, note pinned to his chest:
Send him home when I feel better.

Pain changes us and everything we touch.

Self-Portrait as Cannibal

I know my dog would eat my corpse
rather than starve, though I'd like
to think that first he'd nudge my hands,
lick my face and howl. But if no one
came, eventually he'd have to eat,
obey the voice that said *Survive.*
Afterward, he might be put down
or up for adoption, his new owners
made aware of what he'd done.

Stories of human cannibalism—
the Donner party, airplane crashes
in the wilderness, sailors adrift in open boats—
usually begin when the first person dies
of natural causes and someone argues,
Why let good meat go to waste?
The others slowly, shamefully agree,
giving in because once meat is off
the bone, it could be from anything.
If no one else dies soon enough, debate
begins: Should they draw lots to assign
the sacrifice or starve and wait?

I don't go anywhere without granola bars
shoved in my purse, wrappers crackling
against my keys. But if I was stranded,
starving, if all I had to eat was human flesh,

would I nobly refuse, balk but then surrender,
pray or puke as I reached for my share?
Would I agree to sacrifice myself,
let what was left of me keep them alive?
And if I survived, would I ever speak of what
we'd done, who held the knife and who
the fork, how sweet or bitter the taste?
Would I admit what I'd become?

Instructions for Surviving Slow Apocalypse

In these days of falling ash, it's best to keep
a blanket handy, the bathtub filled with water,

a bucket within reach. The TV says too much.
Listen to the radio instead, especially AM,

low voices pricing hay and feeder cattle.
If you have to breathe in smoke, be sure

to do it slowly. Sore throats are normal
in the morning and late afternoon. If the church

is locked, you can worship Him outdoors,
though the singing may sound hollow.

Stores will run out of staples—bottled water,
batteries and soup—but there will always

be something to buy. Long-lost friends
may call too late at night, their voices blurred

by vodka and sad songs. Be gracious if you can.
Otherwise hang up. Conserve paper,

patience, gasoline. If you begin to panic,
close the blinds. Remember that our days

are always numbered, though we know not how.

Expedition's End

With lines stolen from Michael Pritchett

Bearded, starved, dressed in skins, faces raw
from sun and wind, we begged the first boat
we saw for shirts and whiskey. Our last day
on the river, we passed forty deer gathered
on the bank. We were hungry, close enough
to touch their trembling haunches, but not
a shot was fired. Outside St. Louis, we cheered
at grazing cows—fat, placid, patient.
No one onshore returned our cries.

At the ball given in our honor, we were choked
by our tight collars, dizzied by wine, women
in fine dresses. We'd survived swamps
and fevers, wolves and our own worst natures,
but back in the world, we often felt unwell.
Our tongues were parched and swollen
no matter what we swallowed. Our ears buzzed,
bellies burned, hearts pounded like drums
or buffalo hooves. We couldn't bear
to speak one-tenth of what we'd seen.

We looked to our captains for comfort
or command and found Clark all undone,
Lewis sad and suspicious, hoarding the journals
he'd kept so carefully. We were unfit

to sleep indoors, stand the noise surrounding us,
trust men outside our corps. The wilderness
inside our skulls was vast, starless, hard
to explore. We had no maps or compass,
not a single day's supplies. Unarmed,
we each set off alone, unsure of our return.

Radiation Cento

msnbc.com, 4/1/2011

People within twelve miles have been evacuated
They know they've been exposed to lethal doses
This is not uncommon during emergencies
The world's largest cement pumps are being sent

Known as atomic samurai
Some of them expect to die within weeks or months
If necessary to save the nation
But I think this will not save him

Residents within nineteen miles have been asked to leave
They'll be too hot to come back
Soldiers are searching for the dead
Thought to be a risk for various cancers

I have no doubt it's dangerous there
High levels of radiation within twenty-five miles
To entomb the plant, as at Chernobyl
I wish they'd thought about safety before they ruined our lives

Self-Portrait as a Weary God

When I looked on my work and called it good,
there were no people yet, no prayers
for touchdown passes or miracle cures,

green lights all the way to work. I meant
to be loving all the time, forgiving of those
who apologized, who tried to please me

even if their efforts failed. But people ask
for things they don't deserve, assume
I'll rescue them from their own faults

even if they should've asked much sooner,
listened to the warnings I provide.
I spoke to Moses face-to-face but couldn't

keep it up—it takes too long to reason
and reassure, ease suffering I've seen
infinite times. When I set the world

in motion I didn't know how it
would change, how I'd change in response.
I watch the sparrows when they fall,

when they beat their wings in a cat's mouth,
but I don't always intervene. Sometimes
the void I started with seems like

a restful place, but if I silenced them
I'd miss the voices that I made.

Braem Park

Today it was so quiet in the park
behind my house I could hear leaves
falling to the ground. I let the dog
choose where to walk but kept him

on the leash. Twice we turned around
because branches blocked the path.
Twice I tripped over roots, struggled
to stay upright. Sometimes I saw blurs

between the trees—birds, squirrels
or something bigger. The park is like
the woods but not as wild. City workers
clear the paths and repair fences,

empty trash from plastic barrels.
There are so many half-tame deer
that in December, bow-hunting
is allowed within city limits. I thought

about poachers and how unlike a deer
my dog and I should look, how,
if I saw someone armed in the park,
I might not remember what's in season.

The dog led me down a path I'd never
seen before, across a wood-plank bridge
with iron railings, then to the graveled edge
of a creek we didn't cross. If what I felt

was peace—sun shining between
the branches, dried leaves and needles
under my feet, the smell of summer ending
slowly—I didn't take it home with me.

Aftermath

He doesn't know I've put into poems
every awful thought I had when he was sick,
how often I blamed him and not his body,
wanted the hospital to keep him longer,
wanted his doctors to expect less of me.
When I said to friends, *I can't go on
like this,* I liked being told I didn't have to
visit the hospital twice a day, change
his dressings when he came home,
give up my life for his. I was not a saint.
I was angry, exhausted, said sad
or nasty things because I could,
because I lived in two worlds—the one
in which I taught and went to meetings,
and the one at home where blood
got on the walls, where I picked fights
with my sick husband to prove I suffered, too.

Two years later, we moved to a town
where no one but my husband's doctor knew
how sick he'd been. I wanted to tell.
Instead I carved out poems. *You write
like you're doing surgery,* a colleague said.
I didn't say how right she was,
how much I worry this will break
my marriage: he wants to pretend
it never happened, or that it did and then
it ended. I write about what isn't over,
things we've lost and can't recover.

Carrie Shipers's poems have appeared in *Alaska Quarterly Review, Crab Orchard Review, Connecticut Review, New England Review, North American Review,* and *Prairie Schooner,* among other journals. She is the author of *Ordinary Mourning* (ABZ Press, 2010) and the chapbooks *Ghost-Writing* (Pudding House, 2007) and *Rescue Conditions* (Slipstream Press, 2008).

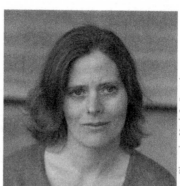

Photo by Kyah Jo Stangl

   Cause for Concern is the winner of the 2014 Able Muse Book Award.

ALSO FROM ABLE MUSE PRESS

William Baer, *Times Square and Other Stories*

Melissa Balmain, *Walking in on People – Poems*

Ben Berman, *Strange Borderlands – Poems*

Michael Cantor, *Life in the Second Circle – Poems*

Catherine Chandler, *Lines of Flight – Poems*

William Conelly, *Uncontested Grounds – Poems*

Maryann Corbett,
    Credo for the Checkout Line in Winter – Poems

John Philip Drury, *Sea Level Rising – Poems*

D.R. Goodman, *Greed: A Confession – Poems*

Margaret Ann Griffiths,
    Grasshopper – The Poetry of M A Griffiths

Jan D. Hodge, *Taking Shape – carmina figurata*

Ellen Kaufman, *House Music – Poems*

Carol Light, *Heaven from Steam – Poems*

April Lindner, *This Bed Our Bodies Shaped –
    Poems*

Martin McGovern, *Bad Fame – Poems*

Jeredith Merrin, *Cup – Poems*

Richard Newman,
    All the Wasted Beauty of the World – Poems

Frank Osen, *Virtue, Big as Sin – Poems*

Alexander Pepple (Editor), *Able Muse Anthology*

Alexander Pepple (Editor),
    Able Muse – a review of poetry, prose & art
    (semiannual issues, Winter 2010 onward)

James Pollock, *Sailing to Babylon – Poems*

Aaron Poochigian, *The Cosmic Purr – Poems*

John Ridland,
    Sir Gawain and the Green Knight – Translation

Stephen Scaer, *Pumpkin Chucking – Poems*

Hollis Seamon, *Corporeality – Stories*

Matthew Buckley Smith,
    Dirge for an Imaginary World – Poems

Barbara Ellen Sorensen,
    Compositions of the Dead Playing Flutes – Poems

Wendy Videlock, *Slingshots and Love Plums –
    Poems*

Wendy Videlock, *The Dark Gnu and Other Poems*

Wendy Videlock, *Nevertheless – Poems*

Richard Wakefield, *A Vertical Mile – Poems*

Gail White, *Asperity Street – Poems*

Chelsea Woodard, *Vellum – Poems*

www.ablemusepress.com